Your Health Now

How to Build Your Immune System During the Covid-19 Pandemic

Copyright ©2021 Dr. Amaka Nwozo DDS

All rights reserved

No part of this book may be reproduced or utilized in any form or by any means, electronic or mechanical, including photocopying, recording, scanning, or otherwise without prior written permission of the publisher. The only exception is brief quotations in printed reviews.

DISCLAIMER

The information in this book is for informational purposes only and it is not intended to be a substitute for professional medical advice, diagnosis or treatment. Always seek medical advice from your physician or other qualified health care provider before exercising or undertaking a new health care regimen. Do not disregard professional medical advice or delay in seeking it because of something you have read in this book. The author and publisher shall have no liability, for any damages, loss, injury, or negative consequences whatsoever suffered as a result of your reliance on the information contained in this book.

Table of Contents

Introduction

Chapter 1: The COVID-19 Pandemic

Chapter 2: Vital Vitamins

Chapter 3: Miraculous Minerals

Chapter 4: The Importance of Superfoods

Chapter 5: Coping with Stress during the Pandemic

Conclusion

About The Author

Introduction

The COVID-19 pandemic has claimed more than 1.9 million lives worldwide to date.
We're going through very difficult times now due to the COVID-19 pandemic. I'll be sharing up-to-date information on COVID-19, the vaccines and how we can enhance our immune systems with superfoods and specific immune system boosting supplements.
Visit us at mindbodyslim.com for more information.

Chapter 1

The Covid-19 Pandemic

Coronavirus disease 2019 (COVID-19) is an infectious disease caused by severe acute respiratory syndrome coronavirus 2 (SARS-CoV-2). Coronavirus disease 2019 (COVID-19) is caused by severe acute respiratory syndrome coronavirus 2 (SARS-CoV-2).
It was identified in December 2019 in Wuhan, China. The pandemic is ongoing and as of today, January 1, 2021, there are more than 90 million cases have been reported across 188 countries and territories. There have been more than 1.9 million deaths and more than 50 million people have recovered worldwide.

How COVID-19 Spreads

COVID-19 spreads when people are physically close to one another and it spreads by droplets in the air. It is very highly contagious and very deadly.

Symptoms

Most of the people infected with Covid-19 don't experience symptoms but for those that do experience fever, cough, fatigue, shortness of breath, loss of taste or smell.

The usual onset is 2–14 days (typically 5). Common symptoms include fever, cough, fatigue, breathing difficulties, and loss of smell and taste but while most people have mild symptoms, some people develop complications. These can be respiratory distress syndrome, multi-organ failure, septic shock and blood clots.

Preventing COVID-19 Infection

Social distancing, washing hands for 20 minutes, wearing masks and face shields can help prevent you from getting COVID-19. People with underlying conditions like asthma, hypertension, obesity, heart disease, cancer fare far worse than those that don't have them.

Three Powerful Vaccines

There are three leading coronavirus vaccines that have been developed to prevent coronavirus infection. The vaccines are made by 3 different companies. One vaccine was developed by the pharmaceutical Pfizer and its German partner BioNTech. The second vaccine was developed by the biotechnology firm Moderna, in partnership with the National Institute of Allergy and Infectious Diseases. The third is from the University of Oxford and its partner AstraZeneca.
Pfizer was given emergency use authorization to the nation's first coronavirus vaccine.

On December 11, 2020, the FDA issued the first emergency use authorization (EUA) for the Pfizer vaccine for the prevention of covid-19 in individuals 16 years of age and older.
On December 14, 2020 the first Pfizer vaccine shots were given in the United States of America.

Three leading coronavirus vaccines are demonstrating strong evidence that they can prevent coronavirus infection. The vaccines are made by 3 different companies. One vaccine was developed by the pharmaceutical Pfizer and its German partner BioNTech. The second vaccine was developed by the biotechnology firm Moderna, in partnership with the National Institute of Allergy and Infectious Diseases. The third is from the University of Oxford and its partner AstraZeneca.
Pfizer was given emergency use authorization to the nation's first coronavirus vaccine.

On December 11, 2020, the FDA issued the first emergency use authorization (EUA) for the Pfizer vaccine for the prevention of coronavirus disease 2019 (COVID-19) caused by severe acute respiratory syndrome coronavirus 2 (SARS-CoV-2).
On December 14, 2020 the first Pfizer vaccine shots were given in the United States of America.
On December 18, 2020, the FDA issued an emergency use authorization (EUA) for the second vaccine for the prevention of coronavirus. The emergency use authorization allows the Moderna

COVID-19 Vaccine to be distributed in the U.S for use in individuals 18 years of age and older.
There are two doses of each authorized vaccine given at specified intervals.
For the Pfizer BioNTech COVID-19 vaccine, the interval is 21 days between the first and second dose.
For the Moderna COVID-19 vaccine, the interval is 28 days between the first and second dose.

COVID-19 Rollout Plan

In the United States, vaccine supplies are limited therefore states are making the vaccine available in phases based on the latest recommendations from the Centers for Disease Control and Prevention (CDC).

Phase 1a: Health care workers fighting COVID-19 and long-term care staff and residents.

Phase 1b: Adults 75 years or older and frontline essential workers.

Phase 2: Adults at high risk for exposure and at increased risk of severe illness.

Phase 3: College, university and high school students 16 or older.

Phase 4: Anyone who wants a COVID-19 vaccine will be able to get one.

Younger children will be vaccinated when the vaccine is approved for them.

Getting to phase 4 may take months so it's still very important to continue to practice social distancing, washing your hands with soap for 20 minutes, wearing your mask and/or face shields. Doing these can help prevent you from getting COVID-19.

We also need to build up our immune systems by eating nutritious food and taking important supplements that will enhance our health during the pandemic. I'll show you how.

Chapter 2

Vital Vitamins

Fruits and vegetables contain amazing micronutrients like phytochemicals, enzymes, vitamins, minerals, antioxidants and macronutrients like carbohydrates, proteins, essential fatty acids and fiber. All these are required to enhance the immune system and enable the body to function at an optimal level.

Micronutrients and Macronutrients

Food is made up of micronutrients and macronutrients. Micronutrients are nutrients required by the body in small amounts and they consist of vitamins, minerals and phytochemicals. Macronutrients are nutrients that are required by the body in large amounts and they include protein, carbohydrates and fats.
Most vitamins and minerals required by the body cannot be produced in the body. They are found in food which makes it important to eat a large variety of food in order for the body to get all the nutrients it requires to function at an optimal level.

Vitamin A

Vitamin A is an organic compound comprised of retinol, retinal, retinoic acid, and provitamin A carotenoids. Vitamin A can be found in two forms in plant and animal. In animals, it is known as retinol and in plants it is the carotenes; alpha-carotene, beta-carotene, gamma-carotene; and the xanthophyll beta-cryptoxanthin. Beta-carotene is the most researched of all the components.
Vitamin A has many functions. It enhances the immune system, bone growth, reproduction, vision and is responsible for healthy hair, skin and teeth. The eye utilizes Vitamin A in the form of retinal.

B Vitamins

B vitamins are water-soluble vitamins essential for cell metabolism. They are coenzymes in many cellular reactions and are involved in cellular functions such as RNA and DNA production, energy production by converting carbohydrates into glucose. Deficiency of B vitamins can lead to fatigue, gastrointestinal issues and skin problems.

Vitamin B1 (Thiamin)

Vitamin B1 plays an important role in energy production through carbohydrate metabolism. It aids nerve and heart function. Vitamin B1 deficiency leads to beri beri and Wernicke-Korsakoff syndrome. Great sources of vitamin B1 are pineapple, tomatoes, flaxseed, meat, liver, eggs and green leafy vegetables.

Vitamin B2 (Riboflavin)

Vitamin B2 is responsible for energy production through fat and protein metabolism. It is also important for growth and development. Vitamin B2 deficiency can cause dermatitis, glossitis and cheilosis. Vitamin B2 is commonly found in almonds, legumes, broccoli, Brussels sprouts, meat, liver, eggs and green leafy vegetables.

Vitamin B3 (Niacin or Nicotinic Acid)

Vitamin B3 is a coenzyme component involved in energy processes. Niacin Deficiency leads to pellagra. Great sources of vitamin B5 are avocados, spirulina, raspberries, meat, sweet potatoes, liver and green leafy vegetables.

Vitamin B5 (Pantothenic acid)

Vitamin B5 plays a vital role in carbohydrate, protein and fat metabolism. Vitamin B5 deficiency is not well characterized in humans. It is commonly found in meat, poultry, liver, legumes, and eggs.

Vitamin B6 (Pyridoxine)

Vitamin B6 plays vital role in protein and glucose metabolism. Deficiency in vitamin B6 is uncommon as it is present in most foods. Vitamin B6 is commonly found in whole grains, bananas, avocados, meat, liver, eggs and green leafy vegetables.

Vitamin B9 (Folic acid)

Vitamin B9 is involved in the formation of genetic materials and maintenance of normal red blood cell production. A deficiency in Folic acid can lead to anemia and neural tube defects. Folic acid can be found in meat, liver, eggs and green leafy vegetables.

Vitamin B12 (Cobalamin)

Vitamin B12 is involved in the formation of genetic materials and red blood cell development. Vitamin B12 deficiency can lead to Pernicious anemia. Vitamin B12 can be found in dairy products, meat, liver, oysters, liver and sardines.

Vitamin C (Ascorbic Acid)

Vitamin C is a water soluble vitamin found in plants and animals. It is an antioxidant that scavenges free radicals in the body. It is also used in the maintenance of connective tissue, cartilage, tendons and bone. It increases the absorption of iron, aids wound healing and muscle regeneration. Vitamin C deficiency can lead to scurvy which is a disease characterized by sore gums, loose teeth, and swollen joints.

Vitamin D

Vitamin D is a fat-soluble vitamin. Two types of Vitamin D exist: Vitamin D3 (cholecalceferol) and Vitamin D2 (ergocalciferol). Vitamins D2 and D3 are found in food and can be obtained from supplements. Vitamin D3 is formed from cholesterol when the skin is exposed to UV rays from the sun.
Research shows that vitamin D deficiency plays a crucial role in cancer development. Scientists believe that 30 percent of cancer deaths could be prevented each year simply by improving the vitamin D levels.

Vitamin E

Vitamin E is a fat soluble vitamin and an antioxidant involved in many enzymatic activities. It is made up of tocopherols and tocotrienols.

Gamma tocopherol is the most common tocopherol occurring naturally in the diet.

Vitamin K

Vitamin K is a fat soluble vitamin that plays a vital role in blood clotting and bone health. Vitamin K deficiency is uncommon in adults because intestinal bacteria is able to produce sufficient amounts. Newborns, however, lack intestinal bacteria because their intestines are sterile. For this reason they are given a vitamin K shot at birth to prevent hemorrhagic disease.

Vitamins	Functions	Conditions Prevented & Treated	Food Sources
Vitamin A	Normal growth and development, maintains integrity of cells such as the gut lining and the skin	Night blindness, infections, colds, poor bone growth, weak enamel	Green leafy vegetables, orange vegetables and fruits
Vitamin B1 (Thiamine)	Energy production	Fatigue, weakness, poor digestion	Vegetables, nuts
Vitamin B2 (Riboflavin)	Growth and development, energy production	Dry skin, dry lips, eczema	Green leafy vegetables
Vitamin B3 (Nicotinic Acid)	Coenzyme component in many biochemical reactions	Anxiety, depression, insomnia, Pellagra	Green leafy vegetables, avocados, sweet potatoes
Vitamin B5 (Pantothenic acid)	Carbohydrate, protein and fat metabolism	Muscle cramps, nausea, weakness	Mushrooms, potatoes, avocados, broccoli.

Vitamins	Functions	Conditions Prevented & Treated	Food Sources
Vitamin B6 (Pyridoxine)	Carbohydrate and protein metabolism	Anemia, cheilosis or stomatitis (cracking of lip borders or corners of mouth)	Green leafy vegetables, orange vegetables and fruits
Vitamin B9 (Folate)	Red blood cell production Synthesis of genetic components	Homocystinemia, megaloblastic anemia, depression. Prevents neural tube defects	Broccoli, spinach, papaya, mangoes, walnuts, lentils
Vitamin B12 (Cobalamin)	Red blood cell production Synthesis of genetic components	Pernicious Anemia, Megaloblastic anemia, progressive peripheral neuropathy	Green leafy vegetables
Vitamin C (Ascorbic Acid)	Antioxidant, connective tissue maintenance, enhances iron absorption, wound healing and muscle regeneration.	Scurvy, bleeding gums, poor wound healing, increased bleeding time, painful glossitis	Green leafy vegetables, avocados, sweet potatoes

Vitamin D (Chalciferol)	Enhances calcium and phosphate absorption. Bone growth and remodeling	Skeletal abnormalities, muscle weakness, painful joints. Prevents rickets and osteomalacia,	Meat, egg yolks
Vitamin E (Tocopherol)	Antioxidant, red blood cell production	Haemolysis, neurologic problems, retinitis pigmentosa, slow healing wounds	Nuts, seeds, cold-presssed vegetable oils, dark green leafy vegetables
Vitamin K	Blood clotting, bone health	Easy bruising, bleeding, increased prothrombin time, weak bones	Asparagus, broccoli, chicken, dark green leafy vegetables, Brussels sprouts

Chapter 3

Miraculous Minerals

Minerals are organic elements required by living organisms for optimal health. They include macro minerals and trace minerals.

Macro minerals

Macro minerals include calcium, phosphorus, potassium, sulfur, sodium, chlorine, and magnesium.
Calcium aids in blood clotting and bone health. It is found in almonds, broccoli, kelp and dates.
Magnesium assists in the absorption of calcium and promotes healthy teeth and bones. Phosphorus promotes strong teeth and bones. Potassium works with sodium to regulate water balance. It also plays a role in muscle contraction and relaxation.
Sodium works with potassium to regulate water balance. It aids in nerve regulation. Chlorine helps regulate electrolyte and fluid balance
Chromium works with insulin to balance blood sugar and regulate the heart. It is found in tomatoes, onions and apples.

Trace minerals

Trace minerals play a catalytic role in enzymes. They include iron, zinc, manganese, copper, cobalt, iodine and selenium.
Iron increases energy and helps transport oxygen in the blood. Zinc improves wound healing and helps regulate nerves.
Manganese promotes strong teeth and bones and helps maintain nerve and tissue function.
Copper plays a role in hemoglobin metabolism and is a component of many enzymes.
Cobalt may help prevent anemia.
Iodine is a component of thyroid hormones that helps regulate basal metabolic rate.
Selenium works as an antioxidant by protecting cells against free radical damage.

Macro minerals	Functions	Conditions Prevented & Treated	Food Sources
Calcium	Blood clotting and promotes bone health	Brittle nails, aching joints. Eczema, heart palpitations, muscle cramps, nervousness	Kale, spinach, almonds, broccoli, kelp, sesame seeds
Magnesium	Absorption of calcium, promotes healthy teeth and bones	Cardiac arrythmias, migraines, hypertension, cardiac arrest, depression	Kale, bananas, pumpkins, nuts
Phosphorus	Promotes bone health	Bone pain, numbness, weakness	Most fruits and vegetables
Potassium	Maintenance of acid base balance, muscle contraction and relaxation	Dry skin, acne, constipation, edema, muscle fatigue, weakness, depression, nervousness	Bananas, almonds and pumpkin seeds

Sodium	Works with potassium to maintain acid base balance	Depression, weakness, fatigue, dehydration, headaches, heart palpitations	Celery, kale, watercress, legumes
Chlorine	Regulates electrolyte and fluid balance	Corrects homeostasis	Salt (Himalayan or Celtic sea salt are best)

Trace Minerals	Function	Conditions Prevented & Treated	Food Sources
Iron	Increases energy and helps transport oxygen in the blood	Anemia, brittle hair, digestive issues, difficulty swallowing, dizziness, fatigue, nervousness	Green leafy vegetables, meat and lentils
Zinc	Improves wound healing and helps regulate nerves	Loss of sense of taste and smell, acne, growth impairment, hair loss, impaired night vision	Pumpkin seeds, nuts and legumes
Manganese	Improves bone health and maintains nerve and tissue function	Atherosclerosis, heart disorders, high cholesterol, memory loss, hearing problems, tremors	Bananas, pumpkin seeds and pineapples

Copper	Collagen formation, hemoglobin metabolism. Copper is a component of many enzymes	Anemia, diarrhea, weakness, skin sores	Vegetables, meat, fish
Cobalt	Prevents anemia	Anemia	Green leafy vegetables, meat, liver
Iodine	Component of thyroid hormone that helps regulate basal metabolic rate	Fatigue, weight gain	Seafood
Selenium	Antioxidant	Cancer, heart diseases, high cholesterol, liver impairment	Brazil nuts, bananas and cashews

Macronutrients

Macronutrients are essential for survival. They are required for the proper functioning of the body and they include protein, carbohydrates and fats.

Macronutrient	Functions	Conditions Prevented & Treated	Food Sources
Protein	Enzymes, antibodies, messengers, structural components, transport and storage of molecules	Weakness, fatigue, malnutrition, diseases	Vegetables, seeds, nuts, sprouted legumes
Carbohydrate Monosaccharides Disaccharides Fiber	Energy	Weakness, fatigue, malnutrition, diseases	Vegetables and fruits

Fat Saturated fats Unsaturated fats (Polyunsaturated and monounsaturated fatty acids)	Fuel, energy, body temperature regulation, insulation	Weakness, fatigue, malnutrition, diseases	Cold pressed vegetable oils, avocados, coconut, nuts, seeds
Trans fats	Trans fats are detrimental to health		Hydrogenated and partially hydrogenated vegetable oils

Benefits of Eating Fruits and Vegetables

- Immune system enhancement: Enzymes, phytonutrients, vitamins, minerals, antioxidants, amino acids essential fatty acids present in vegetables, greens and fruits enhance the immune system. This helps the body to prevent and fight diseases.

- Detoxification: Raw fresh living vegetables and fruit enhance the detoxification of toxins from the body.

- Weight loss: When you eat fresh greens and vegetables that are very low in calories but very high in nutrients and fiber, you are bound to lose weight. Losing weight and permanently keeping it off can help prevent type II diabetes.

- Anti-inflammation: Antioxidants from fresh raw fruits and vegetables remove free radicals in the body preventing inflammation. Some raw foods are more potent in their anti-inflammatory properties than others, for example, ginger and curcumin.

- Anti-microbial: Raw greens and vegetables possess antiviral, antibacterial and antifungal properties that can help the body fight infections.

- Alkalinity: Fruits, leafy greens and vegetables aid the body in maintaining a healthy acid-alkaline balance.

- Improved digestion and elimination: Raw fruits and vegetables contain a lot of water enzymes and fiber. This enhances food digestion and elimination of toxic substances in the form of waste.

- Mental clarity and memory improvement: A diet rich in nutrients and antioxidants helps to destroy free radicals in the body. This has a direct effect on the brain because the oxidative stress in the brain cells is reduced.

- Increased Energy and Vitality: A high amount of enzymes and nutrients are made available to the body through raw food and this gives the body abundant energy and also allows it to heal as well.

- Better Sleep: Protein in food is broken down into amino acids. These amino acids form neurotransmitters that are used in the brain to that help to regulate mood and promote sleep.

- Reduces Disease Risk: When there is an inadequate amount of antioxidants allows free radicals to accumulate in the cells. This can lead to the development of diseases. Antioxidants from raw, living foods like greens and vegetables help decrease the risk of these diseases. The raw food diet is also low in sodium and this could help lower the risk of stroke, heart failure, osteoporosis and kidney disease.

- Longevity: Most vegetables and fruits are low in calories and multiple studies have shown that calorie restriction can increase the lifespan in animals and human beings.

Chapter 4

The Importance of Superfoods

Most vitamins and minerals required by the body cannot be produced in the body. They are found in food which makes it important to eat mostly fresh food because cooking destroys some of the nutrients. Food is made up of micronutrients and macronutrients. Micronutrients are nutrients required by the body in small amounts and they consist of vitamins, minerals and phytochemicals. Macronutrients are nutrients that are required by the body in large amounts and they include protein, carbohydrates and fats.
To be able to obtain all the micronutrients we need, we would need to eat food that contains all the nutrients required and that is not possible because the soil has been depleted of extremely important nutrients due to bad agricultural practices, climate change etc. Dietary supplements include vitamins, minerals, herbs, amino acids, probiotics and enzymes. They are sold in different forms such as tablets, capsules, softgels, gelcaps, powders and liquids.

Benefits of Superfood Supplements

Nutrient dense supplements should not replace complete meals which are necessary for a healthy diet. It is necessary to eat a variety of food and supplement your diet with dietary supplements in order to receive the full benefits of nutrients that will enhance your body's systems to work more efficiently. Nutrient dense supplements can help change your gene expression, enhance your cellular metabolism, improve your gut health, enhance your immune system and so much more.

Amazing Gut Supplements

Enzymes

Enzymes are proteins that catalyze biochemical reactions in the body and are required for the structure, function, and regulation of the tissues and organs in the body.
They also facilitate digestion by breaking down protein, fat, carbohydrates and fiber. This releases nutrients and energy found in the food for use in the body.
The pancreas produces digestive enzymes which are bound to the brush borders of intestinal epithelial cells. They enhance the digestion of food and absorption into the intestinal epithelial cells.
Digestive enzymes include trypsin, chymotrypsin, pepsin, lipase, amylase and protease.

Probiotics

Probiotics are live microorganisms that produce beneficial bacteria that help balance the inner ecosystem and as a result enhance the health of the host. Examples of probiotic bacteria are L. acidophilus, L. ramnosus, L. casei and bifidobacteria.
Probiotics have many functions including providing broad-spectrum anti-microbial activity to protect the

bowel from pathogens. They enhance intestinal barrier function, the absorption of minerals and they help form Vitamin K, Vitamin B12, biotin, and Folate.

Refreshing Omega-3 fatty Acids

Fat is the most important fuel in the body and is essential for function of the human body. It promotes healthy cell function, maintains body temperature, insulates and protects nerves. Fats are sources of essential fatty acids and they enable the absorption and transportation of vitamins A, D, E, and K which are fat-soluble vitamins. This means that their digestion, absorption and transportation depends on fats in the diet. Examples of essential fatty acids are omega 3 fatty acids and omega 6 fatty acids.

Omega-3 fatty acids are important for brain development during the fetal and post-natal periods of life. Decosahexaenoic acid (DHA) is needed for eye development.
They are involved in the synthesis and function of neurotransmitters in the brain.
They synthesize immune system molecules which is necessary for optimal health.

Powerful Antioxidants

Antioxidants are molecules that remove free radicals produced by oxidation reactions in cells. They neutralize free radicals which are produced during metabolism. Antioxidants used by the body include glutathione, vitamin C, Vitamin A, Vitamin E, melatonin, polyphenols, carotenes, CoQ10, lipoic acid. Antioxidants are divided into two groups; water soluble antioxidants such as vitamin C, lipoic acid, glutathione and lipid soluble antioxidants such as carotenes, ubiquinol, vitamin E.

Glutathione (GSH)

Glutathione is the most important antioxidant in the body. It is found in almost all cells and it is formed by three amino acids; glutamic acid, cysteine, and glycine.
Elevated glutathione levels increase cellular antioxidant capacity and decrease oxidative stress. The immune system and antioxidants such as vitamins C and E rely on glutathione to defend the body and prevent disease.
S-acetyl glutathione is the only glutathione supplement that can be absorbed efficiently from the gut. Others are very poorly absorbed so it is best to obtain it from scored tablets of s-acetyl glutathione and food.

Coenzyme Q10 (CoQ10)

Coenzyme Q10 is a compound made by the body and stored in the mitochondria of your cells. It is a very powerful antioxidant that can lower disease risk in heart, brain, lungs, skin and can lower cancer and diabetes risk. Conditions like heart disease, diabetes, brain disorders and cancer have been linked to low levels of CoQ10.

Rich Phytochemicals

Phytochemicals are naturally occurring chemical compounds in plants that provide color, flavor, texture and smell to the plant. They are classified according to their chemical structure. Some phytonutrients also contain chemicals that help protect plants from pests and microorganisms like fungi.
Studies have shown that many phytochemicals are useful in the prevention and treatment of diseases like cancer. Examples of phytochemicals include polyphenols, carotenoids, flavonoids, chlorophyll, glucosinolates, polyphenols, curcuminoids, lignans, stilbenoids, isoflavones, chlorophyll, indoles, protease inhibitors, organosulphurs and terpenes.

Phytochemicals can change the gene expression in cells by regulating the activation of transcription factors such as Nfr2. Examples of phytochemicals that do this include green tea extract, isothiocyanates, sulforaphane and curcumin.

Healing Flavonoids

Flavonoids (or catechins) are members of the polyphenol family and are widely found in fruits and vegetables and often give them their color. Flavonoids are the most abundant polyphenols in our diets with antioxidant activity. Flavonoids are found in celery, cranberries, onions, kale, dark chocolate, broccoli, apples, cherries, berries, tea, red wine or purple grape juice, parsley, soybeans, tomatoes, eggplant, and thyme. Among the important flavonoids are resveratrol, quercetin, and catechins. Research shows that resveratrol may have significant anticancer properties. Wellevate's professional brands manufacture very potent flavonoid supplements which I use as well.

Grape seed extract (GSE)

Grape seed extract (GSE) is derived from grapes and exhibits anti-carcinogenesis because of its cytotoxicity to cancer cells but not to normal cells. GSE is an aromatase inhibitor and has been shown to inhibit aromatase enzymatic activity, aromatase expression and promoter activity. It may lower plasma triglycerides, free fatty acids and lipoproteins in the body. GSE has been shown to have additional properties such as anti-bacterial, anti-viral, anti-inflammatory and anti-allergenic actions. However, a recent study has shown that polyphenols such as GSE and EGCG may inhibit iron absorption therefore it may be important to be cautious when taking them especially pregnant women and children.

Resveratrol

Resveratrol is a polyphenol that is synthesized by grape skins, groundnuts and mulberries in response to injury, ultraviolet (UV) irradiation and fungal attack of these specific plants. It is synthesized in the leaf epidermis and the skin of grapes but not in the flesh.
 Resveratrol is a potent antioxidant and anti-cancer agent.

Quercetin

Quercetin is a plant flavonoid that is most abundant in onions and apples. Quercetin is a powerful antioxidant and heavy metal chelator. Among flavonoids, quercetin was shown to be the most potent inhibitor of COX-2 transcription.

Apigenin

Apigenin is a naturally occurring plant flavone bioflavonoid that is present in leafy plants and vegetables. Research has shown that apigenin has potent anti-cancer effects.

Naringenin

Naringenin is a flavanone, a type of flavonoid, found in all citrus fruits but seen in high amounts in grapefruit, oranges and the skin of tomatoes. It is a free radical scavenger because it reduces oxidative damage to DNA and is therefore an antioxidant. It is also an anti-inflammatory agent, an immune system modulator and it promotes carbohydrate metabolism.

Oleuropein

Oleuropein is a phenolic compound which is found in olive fruit and olive leaves. There are other phenolic compounds found in olive fruit and leaves but oleuropein is the most prominent one that exists. Oleuropein is a powerful antioxidant and it has potent anti-inflammatory, anti-angiogenic, antiviral, antifungal and antibacterial properties and therefore enhances the immune system. It also has anti–cancer properties.

Carotenoids

Carotenoids are orange pigments that are produced by plants and bacteria and are found in almost all colored vegetables especially the yellow and orange ones. Carotenoids include carotene α-carotene, β-carotene, lutein, zeaxanthin, lycopene, β-cryptoxanthin, fucoxanthin, astaxanthin
Humans and animals obtain carotenoids from their diets because they cannot be synthesized in their bodies.
Lutein, astaxanthin and zeaxanthin protect the macula and retina in the eye from damage by UV rays by absorbing them.
Carotenoids such as α-carotene, β-carotene and β-cryptoxanthin are converted to retinol (active form of vitamin A) in the intestine and liver. This conversion occurs in some animals but only 3% of humans can convert it efficiently. Up to 45% of humans are incapable of converting it at all. Animal protein is the best source to obtain retinol. You can get retinol from fish oil and fish.

Glucosinolates

Glucosinolates (GLUs) are compounds found in cruciferous vegetables. Cruciferous vegetables include broccoli, Brussels sprouts, cabbage, cauliflower and kale.
Cruciferous vegetables have the highest concentrations of glucosinolates. There are over 120 GLUs found in cruciferous vegetables some of which include: sinigrin, glucoraphanin, gluconapin, glucoiberin and glucobrassin.

Sulforaphane

Sulforaphane is formed from glucoraphanin which is a major glucosinolate found in high amounts in broccoli/broccoli sprouts. Glucoraphanin is converted to sulforaphane in the body.
It has powerful anti-cancer effects.

Indole-3-carbinol

Indole-3-carbinol is produced by the breakdown of glucobrassicin, Indole-3-carbinol has anticarcinogenic and antioxidant effects.
Indole-3-carbinol reduces cancer risk and incidence by altering estrogen metabolism and other cellular effects.

Garlic

Garlic (Allium sativum) contains organosulfur compounds. Organosulfur compounds are part of the allium family of phytochemicals. Examples are aliin, allicin, Garlic also contains enzymes such as allinase, peroxidases, myrosinase, amino acids, vitamins and minerals.

Garlic is antibacterial, antiviral, antifungal and antiparasitic. It helps to lower blood sugar levels and LDL cholesterol (bad cholesterol).

Aged garlic extract (AGE) is produced by aging garlic that has been shown to block cancer cell growth.

Curcumin (Curcuma longa)

Curcumin is a bright yellow phenolic compound that is derived from the rhizome of Curcuma longa. It is has multiple therapeutic properties such as anticancer, antioxidant, anti-inflammatory, antibacterial, antifungal, antiparasitic, antithrombotic, cardioprotective, neuroprotective, hepatoprotective and hypoglycemic properties.

Curcumin is a very powerful anti-inflammatory agent and a potent chemopreventive agent.

It has been clinically used in cancer prevention and treatment of cancer.

Curcumin is absorbed poorly and has low bioavailability but this can be enhanced by eating curcumin with oil black pepper and quercetin containing food items. Black pepper may also increase breast cancer stem cells sensitivity to curcumin.

Epigallocatechin-3-gallate (EGCG)

EGCG is a natural dietary source of polyphenols, mainly catechins. It is derived from Camelia sinensis or green tea leaves. Catechins are the most active compound found in green tea. The most common catechins are epigallocatechin-3-gallate (EGCG), epicatechin-3-gallate and epicatechin (EC). EGCG has chemopreventive and chemotherapeutic activity against cancer. Its polyphenols act at numerous points regulating cancer cell growth, survival, and metastasis. EGCG has been shown to inhibit cancer cell survival. It is also a potent antioxidant, protecting cells against oxidative damage of DNA, lipids and proteins.

Ellagic acid

Pomegranate contains ellagitannin, and ellagic acid (EA).
The potent antioxidant and anti-atherosclerotic activities of pomegranate juice are attributed to its polyphenols including punicalagin.
Pomegranate contains ellagitannin compounds that have shown to reduce estrogen receptor positive (ER+) breast cancer proliferation by risk by inhibiting the enzyme aromatase.

Melatonin

Melatonin is produced by the pineal gland. It regulates circadian rhythm and has antioxidant, anti-aging and immune enhancing properties. The antioxidant property protects the nuclear and mitochondrial DNA. Research has shown that melatonin has anti-cancer properties.

Chapter 5

Coping With Stress during the Covid-19 Pandemic

We all experience it in our lives but it is much worse these days with business closures and job losses due to the COVID-19 pandemic. We really need to learn how to reduce or even eliminate it to be able to function better for ourselves and our loved ones.

People don't experience the same kind of stress. The magnitude, intensity and individual perception of stress determines how it affects us. It's a personal perceived inability to cope in certain situations in our lives.

Stress is unavoidable but it can be managed and to do that you have to find out what's responsible for causing the stress in the first place. You need to know where, why and how the stress is happening in order to find appropriate ways to reduce your stress or even eliminate it.

Sometimes we create stress for ourselves when we don't have to. We know that these are uncertain times and things are tough for a lot of us. Living through a pandemic is very hard especially when you have children and elderly parents to care for. But we need to remember that we really need to

look after ourselves and be healthy so that we can be there for our loved ones.
During this period we should make important lifestyle changes, create great social connections and live life to the fullest. Yes even now. But to live a fulfilled life you need to start by start loving yourself and putting yourself first. No, you're not being selfish. You're being smart because you want to do the right thing for your life and your family. You want to be healthy and present for your family. You are thinking about others but only in the right order because if you don't look after yourself first, you won't be here to help or look after others.

Types of Stress

There are 2 types of stress - acute and chronic stress.
Acute stress is short in duration but chronic occurs over a long period of time. Chronic stress is never good for the human body. It increases oxidative stress in the cells which can lead to health conditions such as anxiety, depression, stroke, heart problems and cancer. Stress also increases acidity in the body which isn't good for the cellular environment either.
The following can help alleviate stress in your life and assist in helping you achieve optimal health.

13 Ways to Reduce Chronic Stress

1. Social Support
It's very important to have a good social support system. Talking to someone you can trust can really help in reducing stress. This has been proven to alleviate stress.

2. Humor
This really does relieve stress. Laughing everyday can help reduce the pressure feels from stress and anxiety.

3. Change of environment
If at all possible, you may need to change jobs or neighborhoods if your source of stress comes from these.

4. Toxic relationships
This may be the source of your stress due to verbal, physical and emotional abuse. Being in constant stress lowers life expectancy. Ending toxic relationships have been shown to significantly reduce stress.

5. Me time
Spending scheduled time by yourself, doing what you love can also help in reducing stress. Spend adequate time doing what you love every day. Give yourself a break and try and look after your needs.

6. **Visualization**
This relaxes your mind because you are visualizing the truth about who you are and that is blessed and able.

7. **Affirmations**
Making affirmations has been shown to decrease stress and provide a relaxed state of mind, helping to boost confidence.

8. **Organization**
Tidying up your house, work desk etc. can go a long way in reducing stress. Put it on your schedule so that you can make sure you do it.

9. **Time management**
Who hasn't been late for class, meetings, Thanksgiving dinner? Lateness can cause unnecessary stress. Make a schedule. Set your alarm. Give yourself sufficient time to plan and get ready.

10. Exercise

Studies show that regular exercise can reduce stress levels. Exercising outdoors is highly encouraged because the fresh air you breathe helps to increase oxygen flow to the brain. Running, biking, swimming and walking are all great exercises that can be done outdoors.

11. Meditation

By meditating, you are resting and rejuvenating your mind. Studies show that this helps to reduce stress levels because you are in a state of mental quietness or you are thinking thoughts of goodness.

12. Yoga

Yoga is a form of exercise that involves stretching and holding those stretches. It has been shown to reduce stress and may be helpful in the management of depression and anxiety.

13. Counseling

Through counseling you can get help with finding new ways and additional resources to alleviate your stress.

Follow the above do the best you can, live your truth and have fun while doing it!

Conclusion

The COVID-19 virus is deadly and we need to do what we can to ensure that we never get infected with the virus. Get your vaccine shots, practice social distancing and wear your masks until immunity is achieved. Do everything you can to ensure you and your family are safe.

It is impossible for diseases to exist in a body with a very strong immune system but most people don't know whether they have a strong immune system or not. Superfood supplements combined with a diet rich in fresh vegetables and fruits can enhance the immune system and help maintain homeostasis and balance in the body.

Join us at mindbodyslim.com for exclusive offers, tips and recipes!